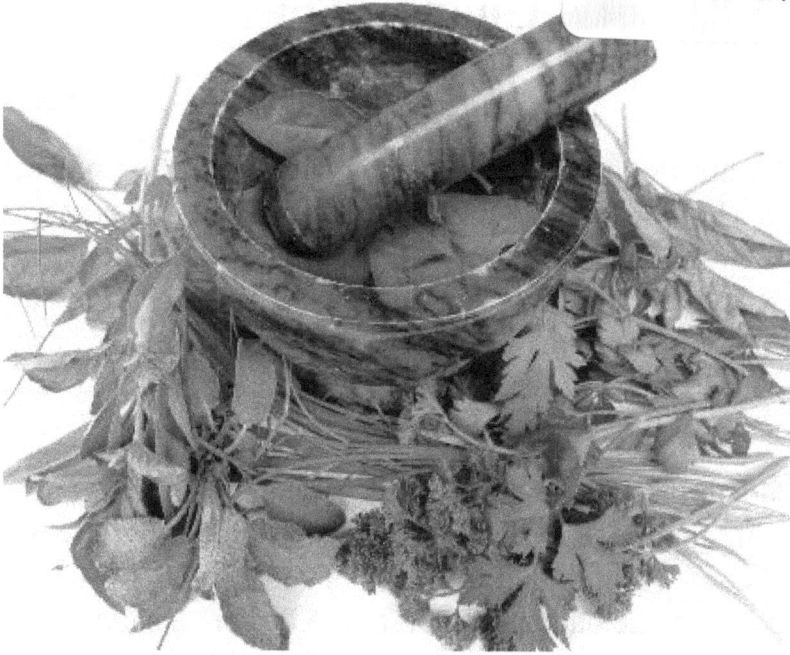

The Lyme Disease Handbook

Michael D. Miller

ISBN 978-0-578-64341-0

1

Chapter One

Introduction

Why am I writing this? Six years ago my health began to fail. My lungs gave out (COPD). Then I got a heart affliction (heart fibulation). I got arthritis, edema in my legs and feet, and blockage in my urinary system. I was a mess. My heart was weak, by lungs were shot, because of my arthritis stiffness I couldn't pick up anything off the floor, and I couldn't pee! Also, I had no energy.

I ended up seeing eight doctors and specialists. But my health continued to decline. I began to think that my time had come (I think that the doctors and specialists did too!). Old age had caught up to me. It got so bad that once, at a restaurant, my wife and I ran into an old friend. After visiting for a while, he quietly told my wife, "Be sure to invite me to Mike's funeral."

I was approaching the end. I got weaker. I went weeks without leaving the house. Then one day, while surfing the Internet, I saw an article about Lyme Disease. It described some of the symptoms of Lyme Disease. They matched my symptoms. The article also explained that Lyme Disease would sometimes mimic diseases such as heart and lung failure. Wow, in a few minutes, my life was changed.

The article explained that Lyme Disease was very difficult for doctors to diagnose. The article also explained that herbal medicines were one of the most effective treatments for Lyme Disease. This elated me, because I had become somewhat of an herbal medicine expert. You see, twenty years earlier, I had helped to pioneer the widespread acceptance of an herbal treatment for cancer called Essiac Tea. I marketed a brand of this herbal tea on the Internet, and we sold this tea worldwide (www.remedies.net). I had written "The Essiac Handbook" which distributed over a million copies worldwide.

So I was well prepared to try out some herbal preparations to see if I had Lyme Disease. As you can guess, I did. My body responded almost immediately, and my symptoms are now gone.

When I checked the Internet, I found that there are almost no herbal or other alternative treatments available for Lyme Disease. So, once again, I am going to be a pioneer. I am going to tell people about Lyme Disease (with this handbook), I am going to tell them how to heal their Lyme Disease, and I am going to prepare and sell a reasonably priced and effective herbal remedy for Lyme Disease.

So I am forewarning you, at the end of this handbook, I will be trying to sell you my herbal tea remedy for Lyme Disease. Or you can make your own tea. I'll tell you how. But the important thing is for you to get healthy.

Background

Lyme disease is a complicated infection that is caused by a bacteria that enters your body from a tick bite. The tick passes into your body a bacteria known as borrelia burgdorferi. This is the bacteria that makes you sick, it is not the tick. So to heal yourself you have to defeat the infection from the bacteria (borrelia burgdorferi).

Overall, up to 300,000 Americans are diagnosed with Lyme disease every year. Thirty percent of them are not cured by their doctor. The antibiotics that they were prescribed didn't work. They are left to suffer years of debilitating pain and suffering. It is to them that I am writing this handbook. We are not in this alone.

Lyme disease symptoms can start with flulike symptoms, headaches, muscle and joint pain. Over time, the symptoms can continue to worsen and turn into a long-lived inflammatory response that is similar to an autoimmune illness.

It's important to understand that although Lyme disease originates from a tick bite, the disease arises due to a bacteria. Two people who are both bitten by the same tick carrying the bacteria that causes Lyme disease can respond very differently. This makes diagnosing the disease difficult. It is also why preventing and treating Lyme disease symptoms by maintaining a healthy immune system is important.

Lyme Disease Symptoms and Causes

The most common Lyme Disease symptoms from the Borrelia burgdorferi bacteria spread throughout the body and cause a series of autoimmune-like reactions.

Research done by the Department of Rheumatology at University of Würzburg in Germany shows that symptoms of Lyme disease are far-reaching and commonly affect the skin, heart, joints and nervous system. Symptoms and signs include:

1. A temporary (acute) "buttery" skin rash that appears where the tick bite occurred (called erythema migrans). Sometimes you may develop a rash shaped like a bull's eye that appears as a red ring around a clear area with a red center. The CDC reports that around 70 percent of Lyme disease patients develop this rash.
2. Flu-like symptoms, especially shortly after being infected. These include

a fever, trouble sleeping, neck pain, fatigue, chills, sweats and muscle aches.

3. Poor sleep, chronic fatigue and lethargy.
4. Digestive issues, including nausea and loss of appetite
5. Achiness and joint pains. The CDC has found that around 30 percent of

Lyme patients develop symptoms of arthritis. Long-term many people experience mood changes, included increased depression and fatigue. Cognitive changes are also a long-term symptom and include forgetfulness, headaches, brain fog, misplacing things and trouble concentrating.

The "REAL" Cause of Lyme Disease:

As mentioned above, Lyme disease is triggered by an infection caused by a tick bite, but there's much more to Lyme disease than that. I believe the real cause of chronic Lyme disease - meaning the type that cannot be effectively treated using antibiotics and lasts for more than six months — is related to these four things:
1. Weakened immunity
2. Inhibited cellular function and protection
3. Systemic bacterial infection
4. Environmental factors including exposure to mold and parasites.

Someone struggling with Lyme disease may have all of these 4 issues, or only one. Some people are able to overcome Lyme disease much more easily than others. Post Lyme Disease Syndrome (PLDS) is how many doctors refer to the condition once it becomes chronic and continues to cause ongoing symptoms for many months, or even years. These patients do not respond to conventional treatments and can experience significant hardships, so much so that their quality of life is reduced due to Lyme disease.

According to medical experts, there might be hundreds of thousands of people who have Lyme disease and don't even know they require Lyme disease treatment. According to Columbia University Medical Center, not everyone who tests positive for the bacteria that causes Lyme will experience Lyme symptoms.

Conventional Lyme Disease Treatment

Healthcare providers often have difficulty diagnosing Lyme disease because many of its symptoms are similar to those of other infectious or autoimmune illnesses, such as the flu, arthritis or lupus. Several tests are now available for diagnosing Lyme disease, although widespread knowledge of these tests is lacking, and some consider these tests unreliable.

Once Lyme is diagnosed, the most common conventional Lyme disease treatment utilized today is prescription antibiotics. The CDC reports that the majority of people can overcome Lyme disease after receiving a course of antibiotics for several weeks. The most common antibiotic treatment for Lyme infection is a combination of amoxicillin, cefuroxime axetil or doxycycline antibiotics taken for 2 to4 weeks.

However, not everyone will respond well to these antibiotics, including those with infections that have spread through the central nervous system. The National Institute of Allergy & Infectious Disease reports that the sooner treatment begins after Lyme infection, the quicker and more complete the recovery will likely be — so people who wait a while before being diagnosed might not react positively to antibiotics.

Antibiotics treat a small part of Lyme disease (the actual infection) but not the entire condition and series of symptoms. Plus, antibiotics can cause side effects and can't always be used in pregnant women or those who are allergic/reactive.

Antibiotics can weaken the immune system over time by negatively altering gut bacteria, especially if they are used for an extended length of time. They kill not only harmful bacteria, but good bacteria that we need for strong immunity, too. This means that antibiotics can possibly make Lyme disease bacteria spread even more and worsen in some people.

Experts generally recommend that the best defense against Lyme Disease is to have a strong and healthy immune system.

This handbook is, in general, written for those people who may have contracted the disease, and have not been helped by antibiotic treatment. This was the condition that I found myself in, and it is why I wrote this handbook. What I learned is that a strong herbal treatment protocol with get rid of your Lyme Disease. There are a number of natural herbs that effectively kill the borrelia burgdorferi bacteria. This is how I got rid of my Lyme Disease. So I now offer my experience to you.

Chapter Two

Effective Lyme Disease Herbs

In this chapter I will describe the herbs that I have found effective to destroy the Lyme Disease bacteria (borrelia burgdorferi).

Cat's Claw

A number of forward-thinking doctors have advanced effective protocols for the treatment of lyme disease. In examining these treatments, it is interesting to note that every one of these doctors recommends the use of the herb "Cat's Claw" as part of their treatment. So let's take a look at this herb:

Lyme and other tick-borne illnesses come with a host of debilitating symptoms. Over time this can lead to serious neurological and cognitive problems.

These illnesses are notoriously difficult to treat, and they can greatly diminish the quality of life. Any herbs that can make a dent in these symptoms should be considered. *Uncaria tomentosa*, better known as cat's claw, appears to fit the bill.

Cat's claw is a plant indigenous to the Amazon rain forest and other tropical
areas of South and Central America. It goes by the Spanish name "uña de gato," (cat's claw) because of a

hook-like thorn that grows along the vine and resembles a cat's claw.

The use of cat's claw for medicinal purposes dates back at least as far as the Inca civilization, where it was used as an anti-inflammatory to fight viral infections, and also to stimulate the immune system. Cat's claw remains a sacred plant among several indigenous Peruvian and Amazonian tribes.

A review of antiviral and immunomodulating properties of plants native to the
Peruvian rainforest noted, "From the perspective of ethnobotany, the higher a
plant's status among native peoples, the more potent it often proves to be
medicinally."

Cat's claw preparations are made from the plant's roots and bark,
which are crushed and made into a tea. In general, studies indicate cat's claw may stimulate the immune system, help relax smooth muscles (including the intestines), dilate blood vessels, and act as a diuretic.

However, specifically for lyme disease, promising research shows that cat's claw is effective. Cat's claw is shown to kill and reduce both spirochetes and rounded forms of the Lyme transmitting organism (*Borrelia burgdorferi*).

In one study of 28 patients with advanced Lyme, it was determined that cat's claw was a powerful intervention for Lyme Disease. Each subject had had the disease for over 10 years, and had experienced progressive deterioration of their condition. They had little to no clinical improvement with repeated doses and long-term use of antibiotics. The study ran for 26 weeks, during which subjects in the control group continued treatment with antibiotics and/or symptomatic medications in accordance with their treatment protocol.

In the test group, all prescription antibiotics were discontinued. They were then given a dosage of 1800mg of cat's claw, given 3 times daily. This dose and supportive remedies were continued for 10 weeks. Then only cat's claw was given for another 16 weeks.

By the end of the study, cat's claw group experienced great improvements. Their symptoms were greatly reduced. (Symptoms included fatigue, joint pain, muscle pain, headache, peripheral neuropathy, sleep disturbances, memory impairment and cognitive dysfunction, digestive disturbances and more.)

The overall results with regard to improving the conditions of the people tested led the researchers to write that cat's claw "is a safe and efficient method for improving the health and quality of life in patients with Chronic borreliosis, and surpasses the effectiveness of standard antibiotics for the treatment of this condition."

Note: The above mentioned was conducted by Amy Berger, MS, CNS. A google search on the Internet will provide any further details of her study that you may wish to check out. There is a wealth of researched documentation out there about Cat's Claw as an effective treatment for Lyme Disease, all available to any Internet researcher (such as yourself).

Garlic as a Lyme Disease fighter

I consider myself somewhat of an expert on herbal remedies. Therefore I know that garlic is, in general, a good remedy for just about everything. It kills infections, it kills parasites, it builds the immune system, etc. I was not surprised therefore to discover that garlic is also good at fighting Lyme Disease.

So let's take a look at garlic as Lyme fighter:

There was a recent study announced by John Hopkins University that said:

LABORATORY STUDY HINTS THAT PLANT COMPOUNDS MAY BE BETTER THAN CURRENT ANTIBIOTICS AT TREATING PERSISTENT LYME BACTERIA AND ASSOCIATED SYMPTOMS

The study reported that garlic and several other common herbs and medicinal plants show strong activity against the bacterium that causes Lyme disease. Garlic may be especially useful in alleviating Lyme symptoms that persist despite standard antibiotic treatment, the study also suggests.

The study, published October 16 in the journal **"Antibiotics"**, included lab-dish tests of 35 essential oils—oils that are pressed from plants or their fruits and contain the plant's main fragrance, or "essence." The Bloomberg School researchers found that 10 of these, including oils from garlic cloves, myrrh trees, thyme leaves, cinnamon bark, allspice berries and cumin seeds, showed strong killing activity against dormant and slow-growing "persister" forms of the Lyme disease bacterium.

"We found that garlic and other essential oils were even better at killing the 'persister' forms of Lyme bacteria than standard Lyme antibiotics," says study senior author Ying Zhang, MD, PhD, professor in the Department of Molecular Microbiology and Immunology at the Bloomberg School.

There are an estimated 300,000 new cases of Lyme disease each year in the United States. Standard treatment with doxycycline or an alternative **antibiotic** for a few weeks usually clears the infection and resolves symptoms. However, about 30 percent of patients report

13

persistent symptoms including fatigue and joint pain—
often termed "persistent Lyme infection" or "post-
treatment Lyme disease syndrome" (PTLDS) that in
some cases can last for months or years. The cause of this
lingering syndrome isn't known. But it is known that
cultures of Lyme disease bacteria, Borrelia burgdorferi,
can enter a so-called stationary phase in which many of
the cells divide slowly or not at all. The slow-dividing or
dormant cells are "persister" cells, which can form
naturally under nutrient starvation or stress conditions,
and are more resistant to antibiotics. Some researchers
have sought other drugs or medicinal compounds that can
kill persister Lyme bacteria in the hope that these
compounds can be used to treat people with persistent
Lyme symptoms.

Zhang and his laboratory have been at the forefront of
these efforts. In 2014, his lab screened FDA-approved
drugs for activity against persister Lyme bacteria and
found many candidates including daptomycin (used to
treat MRSA) that had better activity than the current
Lyme antibiotics. In 2015, they reported that a three-
antibiotic combination—doxycycline, cefoperazone and
daptomycin—reliably killed Lyme persister bacteria in
lab dish tests. In a 2017 study they found that essential
oils killed stationary phase Lyme bacteria even more
potently than daptomycin, the champion among tested
pharmaceuticals.

In the new study Zhang and his team extended their lab-
dish testing to include 35 other essential oils, and found

10 that show significant killing activity against stationary phase Lyme bacteria cultures at concentrations of just one part per thousand. At this concentration, these herbs, derived respectively from garlic bulbs, allspice berries, myrrh trees, spiked ginger lily blossoms and may change fruit successfully killed all stationary phase Lyme bacteria in their culture dishes in seven days, so no bacteria grew back in 21 days.

Further information about these studies can be found at https://globallymealliance.org/news/essential-oils-garlic-herbs-spices-kill-persister-lyme-disease-bacteria/?gclid=EAIaIQobChMIv4vN5LWV5wIVj8DAC

Sarsaparilla

Wild West movies made back in the 1940's often had the Good Guy in his White Hat walk into the local saloon that was full of bad guys. He would walk into the bar, walk up to the bartender, and order a "sarsaparilla". This is how I learned that a sarsaparilla was a non-alcoholic beverage , sweet tasting, that was made from the root of the sarsaparilla vine. It was similar in taste to a root beer or a crème soda.

Eventually drinking sarsaparillas went out of vogue. But now it is known as a powerful herb with several important healing qualities.

Sarsaparilla is a tropical plant. This climbing, woody vine grows deep in the canopy of the rainforest. It's native to South America, Jamaica, the Caribbean, Mexico, Honduras, and the West Indies.

History

For centuries, indigenous people around the world used the root of the sarsaparilla plant for treating joint problems like arthritis, and for healing skin problems like psoriasis, eczema, and dermatitis. The root was also thought to cure leprosy due to its "blood-purifying" properties.

Sarsaparilla was later introduced into European medicine and eventually registered as an herb in the Unites States Pharmacopoeia to treat syphilis.

Sarsaparilla drink

Sarsaparilla is also the common name of a soft drink that was popular in the early 1800s. The drink was used as a home remedy and was often served in bars.

The sarsaparilla soft drink has been described as a similar taste to root beer or birch beer. The drink is still popular in certain Southeast Asian countries, but is no longer common in the United States.

The benefits

Sarsaparilla contains a wealth of plant chemicals thought to have a beneficial effect on the human body. Chemicals known as saponins might help reduce joint pain and skin itching, and also kill bacteria. Other chemicals may be helpful in reducing inflammation and protecting the liver from damage. It is important to note that human studies for these claims are either very old or lacking. The studies referenced below used the individual active components in this plant, individual cell studies, or mice studies. While the results are very intriguing, human studies are needed to support the claims. Here are some benefits:

1. **Arthritis.** Sarsaparilla is a potent anti-inflammatory. This factor makes it also a useful treatment for inflammatory conditions like rheumatoid arthritis and other causes of joint pain and the swelling caused by gout.
2. **Syphilis.** Sarsaparilla has shown activity against harmful bacteria and other microorganisms that have invaded the body. Though it may not work as well as modern day antibiotics and antifungals, it has been used for centuries to treat major illnesses like leprosy and syphilis.
3. **Cancer.** A recent study showed that sarsaparilla had anticancer properties in cell lines of multiple types of cancers and in mice. Preclinical studies

in <u>breast cancer</u> tumors and <u>liver cancer</u> have also shown the antitumor properties of sarsaparilla.

4. **Protecting the liver.** Sarsaparilla has also shown protective effects on the liver. <u>Research</u> conducted in rats with liver damage found that compounds rich in flavonoids from sarsaparilla was able to reverse damage to the liver and help it function at its best.

And now Lyme Disease. Sarsaparilla has been found helpful against infection caused by the borrelia burgdorferi bacteria. Thus it is effectively used to fight Lyme Disease, and it seems that all doctors who prescribe a herbal approach to curing Lyme Disease include sarsaparilla root in their protocols

Oregano

Oregano is a flowering plant that is a member of the mint family. It originally came from the Mediterranean and East European areas. It is widely known as a cooking herb. You probably have some in your kitchen right now. It is treasured for its special flavoring.

Oregano is also used for healing. Oregano offers plenty of medicinal benefits.

The active compounds in oregano can assist in the treatment of diseases such as osteoporosis, diabetes, and even cancer. Traditional medicine revers oregano oil, and homeopaths all over the world regard it for its

18

antimicrobial properties that prevent the spread of disease. Here are some of its benefits: It prevents infection: Studies show the antimicrobial effects of oregano oil in protecting the body from infection. The carvacrol found in oregano essential oil has potent anti-bacterial and anti-viral properties which make it a suitable natural remedy for treating and preventing disease.

Oregano oil or fresh leaf extract helps to alleviate the symptoms of upper respiratory tract infections. Inhaling the medicated steam twice a day may soothe a sore throat, blocked sinus, and reduce levels of fatigue in affected patients.

In addition to the above, oregano is also beneficial as an antioxidant (reducing free radicals in the body), acting as a flu remedy, helping with menstral cramps, assisting against cancer of all kinds, reducing inflammation, killing parasites, and fighting bacterial infections.

Now researchers have discovered that oregano is also an aid in fighting Lyme Disease, and all good Lyme healing protocols recommend oregano.

Ginger

Ginger is one of the most commonly consumed kitchen condiments in the world.

But in addition to its value as a cooking ingredient, ginger has been used for thousands of years for the treatment of numerous ailments, such as colds, nausea, arthritis, migraines, and hypertension. The medicinal, chemical, and pharmacological properties of ginger have been extensively reviewed and studied.

History and Origin of Ginger

Ginger is a member of a plant family that includes cardamom and turmeric. Its spicy aroma is mainly due to presence of ketones, especially the gingerols, which appear to be the primary component of ginger studied in much of the health-related scientific research.

Indians and Chinese are believed to have produced ginger as a tonic root for over 5000 years to treat many ailments, and this plant is now cultivated throughout the humid tropics, with India being the largest producer.

Ginger was used as a flavoring agent long before history was formally recorded. It was an exceedingly important article of trade and was exported from India to the Roman Empire over 2000 years ago, where it was especially valued for its medicinal properties. Ginger continued to be a highly sought after commodity in Europe even after the fall of the Roman Empire, with Arab merchants controlling the trade in ginger and other spices for centuries. In the thirteenth and fourteenth centuries, the value of a pound of ginger was equivalent to the cost of a sheep. By medieval times, it was being imported in preserved form to be used in sweets. Queen Elizabeth I of England is credited with the invention of the gingerbread man, which became a popular Christmas treat.

Usage, Preparation and Processing

Ginger is used in numerous forms, including fresh, dried, pickled, preserved, crystallized, candied, and powdered or ground. The flavor is somewhat peppery and slightly sweet, with a strong and spicy aroma.

Ginger has been purported to exert a variety of powerful therapeutic and preventive effects and has been used for thousands of years for the treatment of hundreds of ailments from colds to cancer. Like many medicinal herbs, much of the information has been handed down by word of mouth with little controlled scientific evidence to support the numerous claims. However, in the last few years, more organized scientific investigations have focused on the mechanisms and targets of ginger and its various components. The evidence for the effectiveness of ginger as an antioxidant, anti-inflammatory agent, anti-nausea compound, and anticancer agent as well as the protective effect of ginger against other disease conditions are now well established.

The variety of protective effects wielded by ginger.

Ginger is a great healing agent because of its antioxidant properties.

(Ginger root contains a very high level of antioxidants, surpassed only by pomegranate and some types of berries.

One of the many health claims attributed to ginger is its purported ability to decrease inflammation, swelling, and pain. Ginger has also been suggested to be effective against osteoarthritis, and rheumatism.

We believe that it is ginger's anti-inflammation qualities that make it an effective addition to our herbs that conquer Lyme Disease.

Thyme

Thyme is a Mediterranean herb with dietary, medicinal, and ornamental uses. The flowers, leaves, and oil of thyme have been used since antiquity to treat a range of symptoms and complaints.

These include diarrhea, stomach ache, arthritis, and sore throat. Also, high blood pressure, foodborne bacterial infections, colon cancer, breast cancer, yeast infection, skin blemishes, and acne.

History: The history of thyme is interesting. People have used thyme throughout history. For example, the ancient Egyptians used thyme as an embalming fluid. In ancient Greece, they used thyme as an incense in temples and added it to bathwater. The Romans used thyme as a flavoring for cheese and alcoholic beverages. They are also supposedly offered it as a cure people for who were melancholic or shy. The Roman army introduced thyme to the British Isles when they conquered the land.

Hippocrates, who lived around 460 BCE to 370 BCE and is known today as "the father of Western medicine," recommended thyme for respiratory diseases and conditions. People grew thyme in gardens and gathered it in the countryside.

When the Black Death took hold of Europe in the 1340s, people would wear posies of thyme for their protection.

Scientific research has shown thyme to have a range of medicinal properties that modern people can put to beneficial use. Now it is found helpful in dealing with Lyme Disease.

Myrrh

When Jesus was born, the three visiting magi brought him gifts of gold, frankincense and myrrh. We all remember this story. But few of us know what myrrh is.

Myrrh is a reddish-brown dried sap from a thorny tree that is native to northeastern Africa and southwest Asia. The tree only grows in a few isolated desert locations. Myrrh was given to Jesus as a special present because it was a very expensive and rare item, very valuable at the time. It was with great difficulty harvested from these very isolated desert locations.

Myrrh is still occasionally used. Myrrh has long been used in traditional Chinese medicine and ayurvedic medicine. It has also been found to have powerful healing abilities, especially for pain, infections, and skin sores.

Here is why we use myrrh: It kills harmful bacteria. Ancient Egyptians used myrrh and other essential oils to embalm mummies, as the oils not only provide a nice scent but also slow decay. Scientists now know this is because the oils kill bacteria and other microbes. Additionally, in Biblical times, myrrh incense and frankincense was burned in places of worship to help purify the air and prevent the spread of contagious diseases, including those caused by bacteria.

In one test-tube study, myrrh oil at a low dilution of 0.1% killed all dormant Lyme disease bacteria, which can persist in some people after antibiotic treatment and continue to cause illness. Thus it is, because of its powerful effect against bacteria, that myrrh as made the list of recommended assist against Lyme Disease.

Chapter Three

Curing My Lyme Disease

When I first read the Internet article that told me that I perhaps had Lyme Disease, I quickly did Internet research on the subject. Then I put together a list of seven herbs that I would put in a tea. I bought the herbs.

Then I made the tea. AAgghh! It tasted terrible. I experimented with several flavorings to mask the terrible taste (chicken flavoring, hyacinth, jasmine, raspberry, stevia, etc.). Nothing worked. Then I tried honey. Aha! It worked fine. I found that maple syrup worked well also. So now, after brewing a cup of the tea, I recommend adding two to three teaspoons of honey or maple syrup as a sweetener. Sweeten to taste.

I drank the tea, twice daily. I experienced almost immediate relief from my health symptoms. I had more energy, my arthritic pain decreased, my lungs got stronger, and I felt better. Getting back to full strength takes a while longer, but my mending was steady and reliable.

I will market my herbal tea on amazon.com. I will call it *"Uncle Mike's Lyme Disease Herbal Tea"*. I will also sell this handbook on amazon.com. Further information is available at www.remedies.net.

I am very proud of my discovery. It has probably saved my life. So now I offer my Lyme Disease Herbal Tea to you and to the world.

This handbook is published by Rideout Publishing, PO Box 1182, Crestone CO 81131.

www.ingramcontent.com/pod-product-compliance
Lightning Source LLC
Chambersburg PA
CBHW070746280326
41934CB00011B/2816